HIGH FIBER FOODS LIST

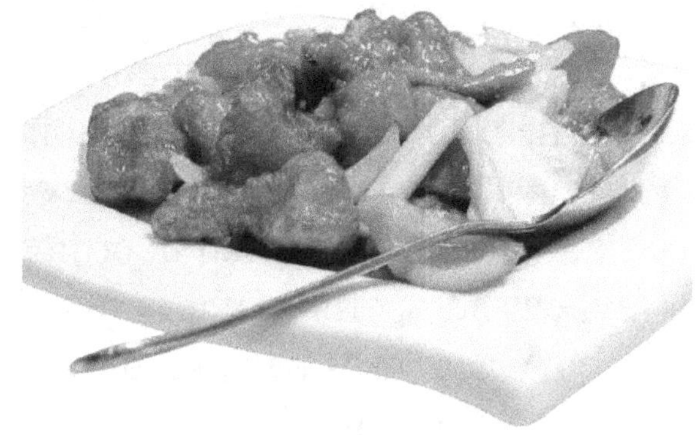

Navigating a High-Fiber Diet: A Complete Compilation of Fibrous Foods Nutrient-Rich Eating Guide.

Felicia O. Pace

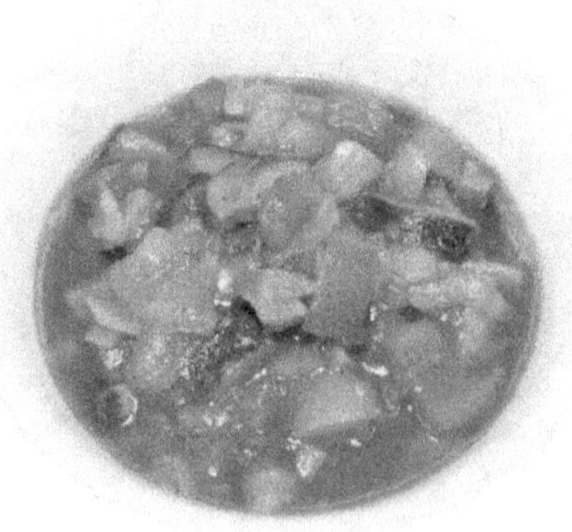

TABLE OF CONTENTS

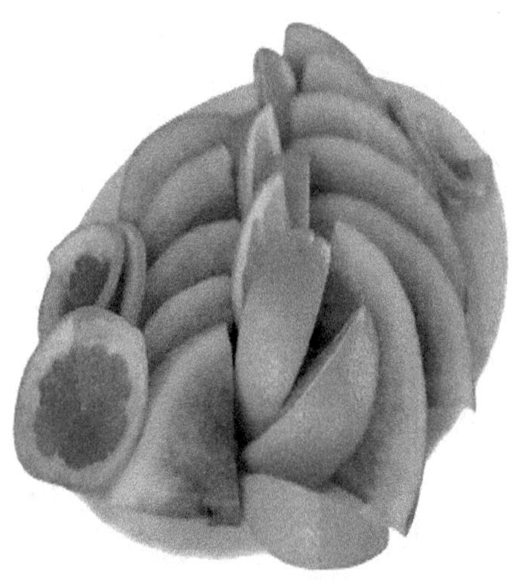

INTRODUCTION

Incorporating high-fiber foods into your diet is a fundamental step toward promoting overall health and well-being. Dietary fiber is a complex carbohydrate found in plant-based foods that offers a multitude of benefits for digestion, heart health, weight management, and more. This high-fiber food list encompasses a diverse range of fruits, vegetables, grains, legumes, nuts, and seeds that can be easily integrated into your daily meals.

Fiber can be classified into two main types: soluble and insoluble. Soluble fiber dissolves in water and forms a gel-like substance, helping to lower cholesterol levels and stabilize blood sugar. Insoluble fiber adds bulk to the stool, aiding in regular bowel movements and supporting digestive health. A balanced diet that includes a variety of high-fiber foods ensures you receive the benefits of both types of fiber.

This high-fiber food list serves as a valuable resource for those seeking to boost their fiber intake. From nutrient-rich vegetables and fruits to whole grains, legumes, and nuts, each entry provides not only substantial fiber content but also a wealth of essential vitamins, minerals, and antioxidants. By diversifying your plate with these high-fiber options, you not only support your digestive system but also contribute to an overall healthier lifestyle.

Whether you're aiming to manage weight, regulate blood sugar, or enhance heart health, this high-fiber food list offers a foundation for creating balanced and nutritious meals. As with any dietary changes, it's advisable to consult with a healthcare professional or a registered dietitian to ensure that your individual nutritional needs are met. Embrace the abundance of fiber-rich foods, and embark on a journey toward better health and vitality.

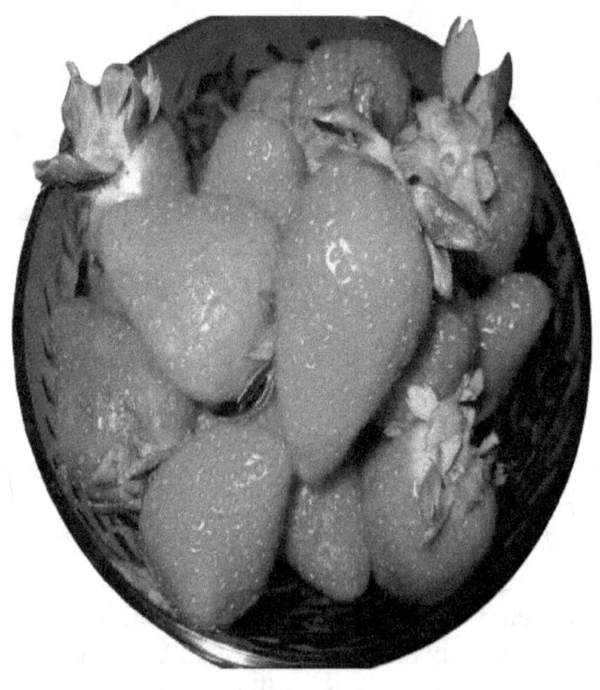

Vegetables

Broccoli:
Recommended Daily Intake: Men - 38 grams, Women - 25 grams
Fiber Content: Approximately 2.4 grams per 1 cup (cooked)
Nutrition: Rich in vitamins C and K, folate, and a good source of antioxidants.

Brussels Sprouts:
Recommended Daily Intake: Men - 38 grams, Women - 25 grams
Fiber Content: Approximately 3.3 grams per 1 cup (cooked)
Nutrition: High in vitamins K and C, as well as containing small amounts of other nutrients.

Carrots:
Recommended Daily Intake: Men - 38 grams, Women - 25 grams
Fiber Content: Approximately 3.6 grams per 1 cup (raw)
Nutrition: Rich in beta-carotene, vitamin K, and potassium.

Spinach:
Recommended Daily Intake: Men - 38 grams, Women - 25 grams
Fiber Content: Approximately 6.7 grams per 1 cup (cooked)

Nutrition: High in iron, calcium, vitamins A and K, and various antioxidants.

Sweet Potatoes:
Recommended Daily Intake: Men - 38 grams, Women - 25 grams
Fiber Content: Approximately 4 grams per 1 medium-sized sweet potato (baked with skin)
Nutrition: Rich in beta-carotene, vitamin C, and manganese.

Artichokes:
Recommended Daily Intake: Men - 38 grams, Women - 25 grams
Fiber Content: Approximately 6.7 grams per 1 medium-sized artichoke (cooked)
Nutrition: Good source of folate, vitamin K, and magnesium.

Cauliflower:
Recommended Daily Intake: Men - 38 grams, Women - 25 grams
Fiber Content: Approximately 2.1 grams per 1 cup (raw)
Nutrition: Contains vitamins C, K, and B6, as well as folate and choline.

Bell Peppers:
Recommended Daily Intake: Men - 38 grams, Women - 25 grams
Fiber Content: Approximately 2.5 grams per 1 cup (raw)
Nutrition: High in vitamin C, A, and potassium.

Cabbage:
Recommended Daily Intake: Men - 38 grams, Women - 25 grams
Fiber Content: Approximately 2.2 grams per 1 cup (raw)
Nutrition: Contains vitamin K, C, and B6, as well as folate and manganese.

Kale:
Recommended Daily Intake: Men - 38 grams, Women - 25 grams
Fiber Content: Approximately 2.6 grams per 1 cup (raw)
Nutrition: Rich in vitamins K, A, and C, along with calcium and antioxidants.

Nuts and Seeds

Chia Seeds:
Recommended Daily Intake: Men - 38 grams, Women - 25 grams
Fiber Content: Approximately 10.6 grams per 1 ounce (about 2 tablespoons)
Nutrition: High in omega-3 fatty acids, protein, and various minerals.

Flaxseeds:
Recommended Daily Intake: Men - 38 grams, Women - 25 grams
Fiber Content: Approximately 7.6 grams per 1 ounce (about 2 tablespoons)
Nutrition: Rich in omega-3 fatty acids, lignans, and antioxidants.

Almonds:
Recommended Daily Intake: Men - 38 grams, Women - 25 grams
Fiber Content: Approximately 3.5 grams per 1 ounce (about 23 almonds)
Nutrition: High in vitamin E, magnesium, and monounsaturated fats.

Pumpkin Seeds (Pepitas):
Recommended Daily Intake: Men - 38 grams, Women - 25 grams
Fiber Content: Approximately 5.2 grams per 1 ounce (about 2 tablespoons)
Nutrition: Good source of iron, magnesium, zinc, and protein.

Sunflower Seeds:
Recommended Daily Intake: Men - 38 grams, Women - 25 grams
Fiber Content: Approximately 3.9 grams per 1 ounce (about 2 tablespoons)
Nutrition: Rich in vitamin E, magnesium, and selenium.

Walnuts:
Recommended Daily Intake: Men - 38 grams, Women - 25 grams
Fiber Content: Approximately 1.9 grams per 1 ounce (about 14 halves)
Nutrition: High in omega-3 fatty acids, antioxidants, and protein.

Pistachios:
Recommended Daily Intake: Men - 38 grams, Women - 25 grams
Fiber Content: Approximately 2.9 grams per 1 ounce (about 49 kernels)
Nutrition: Good source of protein, vitamin B6, and potassium.

Hazelnuts:
Recommended Daily Intake: Men - 38 grams, Women - 25 grams
Fiber Content: Approximately 2.7 grams per 1 ounce (about 21 kernels)
Nutrition: High in vitamin E, magnesium, and monounsaturated fats.

Cashews:
Recommended Daily Intake: Men - 38 grams, Women - 25 grams
Fiber Content: Approximately 1 gram per 1 ounce (about 18 cashews)
Nutrition: Rich in iron, zinc, and monounsaturated fats.

Pecans:
Recommended Daily Intake: Men - 38 grams, Women - 25 grams
Fiber Content: Approximately 2.7 grams per 1 ounce (about 19 halves)
Nutrition: High in antioxidants, manganese, and monounsaturated fats.

Whole grains

Quinoa:
Recommended Daily Intake: Men - 38 grams,
Women - 25 grams
Fiber Content: Approximately 5.2 grams per 1 cup
(cooked)
Nutrition: Good source of protein, iron, magnesium,
and antioxidants.

Oats:
Recommended Daily Intake: Men - 38 grams,
Women - 25 grams
Fiber Content: Approximately 4 grams per 1 cup
(cooked)
Nutrition: Rich in beta-glucans, a type of soluble
fiber, and contains manganese and phosphorus.

Brown Rice:
Recommended Daily Intake: Men - 38 grams,
Women - 25 grams
Fiber Content: Approximately 3.5 grams per 1 cup
(cooked)
Nutrition: Good source of manganese, magnesium,
and selenium.

Barley:
Recommended Daily Intake: Men - 38 grams,
Women - 25 grams
Fiber Content: Approximately 6 grams per 1 cup
(cooked)
Nutrition: Contains beta-glucans and provides
essential nutrients like selenium and copper.

Bulgur:
Recommended Daily Intake: Men - 38 grams, Women - 25 grams
Fiber Content: Approximately 8.2 grams per 1 cup (cooked)
Nutrition: Good source of manganese, magnesium, and iron.

Whole Wheat Pasta:
Recommended Daily Intake: Men - 38 grams, Women - 25 grams
Fiber Content: Approximately 6.3 grams per 1 cup (cooked)
Nutrition: Provides fiber, protein, and various B-vitamins.

Farro:
Recommended Daily Intake: Men - 38 grams, Women - 25 grams
Fiber Content: Approximately 7.9 grams per 1 cup (cooked)
Nutrition: Rich in protein, fiber, and nutrients such as magnesium and zinc.

Millet:
Recommended Daily Intake: Men - 38 grams, Women - 25 grams
Fiber Content: Approximately 2.3 grams per 1 cup (cooked)
Nutrition: Contains antioxidants, magnesium, and other essential minerals.
Freekeh:

Recommended Daily Intake: Men - 38 grams, Women - 25 grams
Fiber Content: Approximately 8.6 grams per 1 cup (cooked)
Nutrition: High in protein, fiber, and various vitamins and minerals.

Amaranth:
Recommended Daily Intake: Men - 38 grams, Women - 25 grams
Fiber Content: Approximately 5.2 grams per 1 cup (cooked)
Nutrition: Rich in protein, iron, and calcium.

Legumes and Beans

Lentils:
Recommended Daily Intake: Men - 38 grams, Women - 25 grams
Fiber Content: Approximately 15.6 grams per 1 cup (cooked)
Nutrition: Rich in protein, folate, iron, and other essential nutrients.

Black Beans:
Recommended Daily Intake: Men - 38 grams, Women - 25 grams
Fiber Content: Approximately 15 grams per 1 cup (cooked)
Nutrition: Good source of protein, iron, potassium, and antioxidants.

Chickpeas (Garbanzo Beans):
Recommended Daily Intake: Men - 38 grams, Women - 25 grams
Fiber Content: Approximately 12.5 grams per 1 cup (cooked)
Nutrition: High in protein, folate, iron, and manganese.

Kidney Beans:
Recommended Daily Intake: Men - 38 grams, Women - 25 grams
Fiber Content: Approximately 11.3 grams per 1 cup (cooked)
Nutrition: Rich in protein, iron, potassium, and antioxidants.

Pinto Beans:
Recommended Daily Intake: Men - 38 grams, Women - 25 grams
Fiber Content: Approximately 15.4 grams per 1 cup (cooked)
Nutrition: Good source of protein, iron, and manganese.

Black-eyed Peas:
Recommended Daily Intake: Men - 38 grams, Women - 25 grams
Fiber Content: Approximately 11.2 grams per 1 cup (cooked)
Nutrition: High in protein, folate, and various vitamins and minerals.

Split Peas:
Recommended Daily Intake: Men - 38 grams, Women - 25 grams
Fiber Content: Approximately 16.3 grams per 1 cup (cooked)
Nutrition: Rich in protein, folate, and iron.

Cannellini Beans:
Recommended Daily Intake: Men - 38 grams, Women - 25 grams
Fiber Content: Approximately 13.1 grams per 1 cup (cooked)
Nutrition: Good source of protein, iron, and potassium.

Adzuki Beans:
Recommended Daily Intake: Men - 38 grams, Women - 25 grams
Fiber Content: Approximately 16.8 grams per 1 cup (cooked)
Nutrition: High in protein, folate, and iron.

Great Northern Beans:
Recommended Daily Intake: Men - 38 grams, Women - 25 grams
Fiber Content: Approximately 12.4 grams per 1 cup (cooked)
Nutrition: Good source of protein, folate, and iron.

Fruits

Raspberries:
Recommended Daily Intake: Men - 38 grams, Women - 25 grams
Fiber Content: Approximately 8 grams per cup (raw)
Nutrition: Rich in vitamin C, manganese, and antioxidants.

Blackberries:
Recommended Daily Intake: Men - 38 grams, Women - 25 grams
Fiber Content: Approximately 7.6 grams per cup (raw)
Nutrition: High in vitamin C, vitamin K, and antioxidants.

Pears:
Recommended Daily Intake: Men - 38 grams, Women - 25 grams
Fiber Content: Approximately 5.5 grams per medium-sized pear (with skin)
Nutrition: Good source of vitamin C, potassium, and antioxidants.

Apples:
Recommended Daily Intake: Men - 38 grams, Women - 25 grams
Fiber Content: Approximately 4.4 grams per medium-sized apple (with skin)
Nutrition: Contains vitamin C, potassium, and various antioxidants.

Avocado:
Recommended Daily Intake: Men - 38 grams, Women - 25 grams
Fiber Content: Approximately 10 grams per cup (sliced)
Nutrition: High in healthy monounsaturated fats, vitamin K, and potassium.

Bananas:
Recommended Daily Intake: Men - 38 grams, Women - 25 grams
Fiber Content: Approximately 3.1 grams per medium-sized banana
Nutrition: Good source of potassium, vitamin C, and vitamin B6.

Strawberries:
Recommended Daily Intake: Men - 38 grams, Women - 25 grams
Fiber Content: Approximately 3 grams per cup (sliced)
Nutrition: High in vitamin C, manganese, and antioxidants.

Guava:
Recommended Daily Intake: Men - 38 grams, Women - 25 grams
Fiber Content: Approximately 9 grams per cup (raw)
Nutrition: Rich in vitamin C, fiber, and antioxidants.

Oranges:
Recommended Daily Intake: Men - 38 grams, Women - 25 grams

Fiber Content: Approximately 4.3 grams per medium-sized orange
Nutrition: High in vitamin C, potassium, and folate.

Kiwi:
Recommended Daily Intake: Men - 38 grams, Women - 25 grams
Fiber Content: Approximately 5.4 grams per cup (sliced)
Nutrition: Rich in vitamin C, vitamin K, and antioxidants.

Cereals

Bran Flakes:
Recommended Daily Intake: Men - 38 grams, Women - 25 grams
Fiber Content: Approximately 7 grams per 3/4 cup serving
Nutrition: Good source of fiber, iron, and various B-vitamins.

Shredded Wheat:
Recommended Daily Intake: Men - 38 grams, Women - 25 grams
Fiber Content: Approximately 6 grams per 2 biscuit serving (without added sugar)
Nutrition: Minimal ingredients, high in fiber, and no added sugars.

Oat Bran Cereal:
Recommended Daily Intake: Men - 38 grams, Women - 25 grams
Fiber Content: Approximately 4 grams per 1/3 cup serving
Nutrition: High in beta-glucans, which can help lower cholesterol.

All-Bran:
Recommended Daily Intake: Men - 38 grams, Women - 25 grams
Fiber Content: Approximately 10 grams per 1/2 cup serving
Nutrition: Excellent source of fiber, low in fat, and contains vitamins and minerals.

Quinoa Flakes Cereal:
Recommended Daily Intake: Men - 38 grams, Women - 25 grams
Fiber Content: Approximately 5 grams per 1/2 cup serving
Nutrition: Provides protein, iron, and a good alternative for those with gluten sensitivity.

Granola with Nuts and Seeds:
Recommended Daily Intake: Men - 38 grams, Women - 25 grams
Fiber Content: Approximately 4 grams per 1/2 cup serving
Nutrition: Rich in healthy fats, protein, and various nutrients. Watch for added sugars.

Multigrain Cereal:
Recommended Daily Intake: Men - 38 grams, Women - 25 grams
Fiber Content: Approximately 5 grams per 1 cup serving
Nutrition: Typically a mix of different grains, providing a variety of nutrients.

High-Fiber Raisin Bran:
Recommended Daily Intake: Men - 38 grams, Women - 25 grams
Fiber Content: Approximately 7 grams per 1 cup serving
Nutrition: Combines fiber from bran with the natural sweetness of raisins.

Honey Nut Fiber Cereal:
Recommended Daily Intake: Men - 38 grams, Women - 25 grams
Fiber Content: Approximately 5 grams per 3/4 cup serving
Nutrition: Provides fiber with the added flavor of honey and nuts. Watch for added sugars.

Whole Grain Puffed Cereal:
Recommended Daily Intake: Men - 38 grams, Women - 25 grams
Fiber Content: Approximately 1 gram per 1 cup serving
Nutrition: Low in sugar and fat, good for those looking for a simple, whole grain option.

Almond Milk:
Recommended Daily Intake: Men - 38 grams, Women - 25 grams
Fiber Content: Approximately 1 gram per cup (unsweetened)
Nutrition: Almond milk is low in calories and can be fortified with vitamins and minerals.

Soy Milk:
Recommended Daily Intake: Men - 38 grams, Women - 25 grams
Fiber Content: Approximately 2 grams per cup (unsweetened)
Nutrition: Soy milk is a good source of plant-based protein and is often fortified with calcium and vitamin D.

Oat Milk:
Recommended Daily Intake: Men - 38 grams, Women - 25 grams
Fiber Content: Approximately 2 grams per cup (unsweetened)
Nutrition: Oat milk is naturally sweet and provides a good source of carbohydrates.

Coconut Milk:
Recommended Daily Intake: Men - 38 grams, Women - 25 grams
Fiber Content: Approximately 0.5 grams per cup (unsweetened)

Nutrition: Coconut milk is rich in healthy fats but may be lower in protein and fiber.

Cashew Milk:

Recommended Daily Intake: Men - 38 grams, Women - 25 grams

Fiber Content: Approximately 0.5 grams per cup (unsweetened)

Nutrition: Cashew milk is creamy and can be a good source of healthy fats.

Rice Milk:

Recommended Daily Intake: Men - 38 grams, Women - 25 grams

Fiber Content: Approximately 0 grams per cup (unsweetened)

Nutrition: Rice milk is often well-tolerated by those with nut or soy allergies but may be lower in protein and fiber.

Flax Milk:

Recommended Daily Intake: Men - 38 grams, Women - 25 grams

Fiber Content: Approximately 1 gram per cup (unsweetened)

Nutrition: Flax milk contains omega-3 fatty acids and can be a good source of ALA.

Hemp Milk:

Recommended Daily Intake: Men - 38 grams, Women - 25 grams

Fiber Content: Approximately 0.5 grams per cup (unsweetened)

Nutrition: Hemp milk provides a balance of omega-3 and omega-6 fatty acids.

Quinoa Milk:
Recommended Daily Intake: Men - 38 grams, Women - 25 grams
Fiber Content: Approximately 1.5 grams per cup (unsweetened)
Nutrition: Quinoa milk is a good source of plant-based protein and can be fortified with vitamins and minerals.

Pea Milk:
Recommended Daily Intake: Men - 38 grams, Women - 25 grams
Fiber Content: Approximately 1 gram per cup (unsweetened)
Nutrition: Pea milk is high in protein and is often fortified with nutrients.

SIMPLE AND DELICIOUS RECIPES

Breakfast Recipes

1. Oatmeal with Berries and Nuts:
Recommended Daily Intake: Men - 38 grams, Women - 25 grams
Fiber Content: Approximately 8 grams per 1 cup (cooked oats)
Nutrition: Oats provide beta-glucans, a soluble fiber, while berries and nuts add antioxidants, vitamins, and healthy fats.

2. Whole Grain Toast with Avocado and Poached Egg:
Recommended Daily Intake: Men - 38 grams, Women - 25 grams
Fiber Content: Approximately 7 grams per two slices of whole grain bread
Nutrition: Avocado offers healthy monounsaturated fats, and the poached egg adds protein and additional nutrients.

3. Greek Yogurt Parfait with Granola and Fruit:
Recommended Daily Intake: Men - 38 grams, Women - 25 grams
Fiber Content: Approximately 6 grams per cup of Greek yogurt (without added sugars)
Nutrition: Greek yogurt provides protein, while granola and fruit contribute fiber, vitamins, and minerals.

4. Chia Seed Pudding with Berries:
Recommended Daily Intake: Men - 38 grams, Women - 25 grams
Fiber Content: Approximately 10 grams per 2 tablespoons of chia seeds (when mixed with liquid)
Nutrition: Chia seeds are rich in omega-3 fatty acids, and berries add antioxidants and vitamins.

5. Whole Grain Pancakes with Maple Syrup and Bananas:
Recommended Daily Intake: Men - 38 grams, Women - 25 grams
Fiber Content: Approximately 3 grams per pancake (using whole grain flour)
Nutrition: Whole grain pancakes offer fiber, and bananas provide potassium and additional fiber.

6. Smoothie with Spinach, Banana, and Flaxseeds:
Recommended Daily Intake: Men - 38 grams, Women - 25 grams
Fiber Content: Approximately 5 grams per cup (when blended with fruits and vegetables)
Nutrition: Spinach adds fiber and nutrients, while flaxseeds contribute omega-3 fatty acids.

7. Vegetable Omelette with Whole Grain Toast:
Recommended Daily Intake: Men - 38 grams, Women - 25 grams
Fiber Content: Approximately 4 grams per two slices of whole grain toast
Nutrition: Vegetables in the omelette provide fiber, vitamins, and minerals, while whole grain toast adds additional fiber.

8. Whole Grain Bagel with Cream Cheese and Smoked Salmon:
Recommended Daily Intake: Men - 38 grams, Women - 25 grams
Fiber Content: Approximately 4 grams per whole grain bagel
Nutrition: Salmon adds omega-3 fatty acids, and whole grain bagel provides fiber.

9. Fruit and Nut Overnight Oats:
Recommended Daily Intake: Men - 38 grams, Women - 25 grams
Fiber Content: Approximately 7 grams per 1 cup (prepared with oats, milk, fruits, and nuts)
Nutrition: Oats and nuts add fiber and nutrients, while fruits provide natural sweetness.

10. Bran Muffins with Greek Yogurt:
- Recommended Daily Intake: Men - 38 grams, Women - 25 grams
- Fiber Content: Approximately 5 grams per muffin (using bran)
- Nutrition: Bran muffins offer fiber, and Greek yogurt provides protein and additional nutrients.

Lunch Recipes

1. Quinoa and Black Bean Salad:
Recommended Daily Intake: Men - 38 grams, Women - 25 grams
Fiber Content: Approximately 15 grams per cup (cooked quinoa and black beans)
Nutrition: Quinoa provides complete protein, and black beans add fiber, protein, and various nutrients.

2. Chickpea and Vegetable Stir-Fry:
Recommended Daily Intake: Men - 38 grams, Women - 25 grams
Fiber Content: Approximately 10 grams per cup (cooked chickpeas and vegetables)
Nutrition: Chickpeas offer protein, and colorful vegetables provide fiber, vitamins, and minerals.

3. Lentil Soup with Whole Grain Bread:
Recommended Daily Intake: Men - 38 grams, Women - 25 grams
Fiber Content: Approximately 14 grams per cup (cooked lentils)
Nutrition: Lentils are rich in protein and fiber, while whole grain bread adds more fiber.

4. Spinach and Feta Stuffed Bell Peppers:
Recommended Daily Intake: Men - 38 grams, Women - 25 grams
Fiber Content: Approximately 7 grams per medium-sized bell pepper

Nutrition: Bell peppers offer fiber and vitamins, and spinach and feta provide additional nutrients.

5. Whole Grain Wrap with Turkey and Hummus:
Recommended Daily Intake: Men - 38 grams, Women - 25 grams
Fiber Content: Approximately 7 grams per whole grain wrap
Nutrition: Turkey adds protein, while hummus and whole grain wrap contribute fiber and healthy fats.

6. Quinoa and Vegetable Buddha Bowl:
Recommended Daily Intake: Men - 38 grams, Women - 25 grams
Fiber Content: Approximately 12 grams per bowl (cooked quinoa and mixed vegetables)
Nutrition: Quinoa provides protein, and a variety of vegetables add fiber, vitamins, and minerals.

7. Black Bean and Sweet Potato Quesadilla:
Recommended Daily Intake: Men - 38 grams, Women - 25 grams
Fiber Content: Approximately 12 grams per quesadilla
Nutrition: Black beans offer fiber and protein, and sweet potatoes provide additional fiber and nutrients.

8. Greek Salad with Chickpea Patties:
Recommended Daily Intake: Men - 38 grams, Women - 25 grams
Fiber Content: Approximately 10 grams per cup (chickpea patties and vegetables)

Nutrition: Chickpea patties add protein and fiber, while the Greek salad provides vitamins and minerals.

9. Brown Rice and Vegetable Sushi Rolls:
Recommended Daily Intake: Men - 38 grams, Women - 25 grams
Fiber Content: Approximately 6 grams per cup (cooked brown rice and vegetables)
Nutrition: Brown rice offers fiber, and vegetables provide additional nutrients.

10. Lentil and Vegetable Curry with Quinoa:
- Recommended Daily Intake: Men - 38 grams, Women - 25 grams
- Fiber Content: Approximately 14 grams per cup (cooked lentils and quinoa)
- Nutrition: Lentils add protein and fiber, while quinoa provides additional protein and nutrients.

Dinner Recipes

1. Chickpea and Vegetable Curry with Brown Rice:
Recommended Daily Intake: Men - 38 grams, Women - 25 grams
Fiber Content: Approximately 12 grams per cup (cooked chickpeas and brown rice)
Nutrition: Chickpeas provide protein and fiber, and brown rice adds additional fiber and nutrients.

2. Spaghetti Squash with Lentil Bolognese:
Recommended Daily Intake: Men - 38 grams, Women - 25 grams
Fiber Content: Approximately 11 grams per cup (cooked lentils and spaghetti squash)
Nutrition: Lentils offer protein and fiber, and spaghetti squash is a low-calorie alternative to pasta.

3. Vegetarian Quinoa and Black Bean Stuffed Peppers:
Recommended Daily Intake: Men - 38 grams, Women - 25 grams
Fiber Content: Approximately 14 grams per cup (cooked quinoa and black beans)
Nutrition: Quinoa provides protein, and black beans add fiber and additional nutrients.

4. Salmon and Quinoa Salad with Avocado Dressing:
Recommended Daily Intake: Men - 38 grams, Women - 25 grams
Fiber Content: Approximately 8 grams per cup (cooked quinoa and vegetables)
Nutrition: Salmon offers omega-3 fatty acids, and quinoa provides protein and fiber. Avocado dressing adds healthy fats.

5. Whole Wheat Pasta with Roasted Vegetables and Pesto:
Recommended Daily Intake: Men - 38 grams, Women - 25 grams
Fiber Content: Approximately 8 grams per cup (cooked whole wheat pasta and vegetables)

Nutrition: Whole wheat pasta adds fiber, and roasted vegetables provide vitamins and minerals. Pesto adds flavor and healthy fats.

6. Black Bean and Vegetable Quesadillas:
Recommended Daily Intake: Men - 38 grams, Women - 25 grams
Fiber Content: Approximately 10 grams per quesadilla
Nutrition: Black beans offer protein and fiber, and vegetables provide additional fiber and nutrients.

7. Stuffed Portobello Mushrooms with Quinoa and Spinach:
Recommended Daily Intake: Men - 38 grams, Women - 25 grams
Fiber Content: Approximately 9 grams per cup (cooked quinoa and spinach)
Nutrition: Quinoa provides protein and fiber, and spinach adds vitamins and minerals.

8. Grilled Chicken and Vegetable Kebabs with Quinoa:
Recommended Daily Intake: Men - 38 grams, Women - 25 grams
Fiber Content: Approximately 7 grams per cup (cooked quinoa and vegetables)
Nutrition: Chicken offers protein, and vegetables provide fiber, vitamins, and minerals.

9. Barley and Mushroom Risotto:
Recommended Daily Intake: Men - 38 grams, Women - 25 grams
Fiber Content: Approximately 8 grams per cup (cooked barley and mushrooms)
Nutrition: Barley adds fiber, and mushrooms provide additional nutrients.

10. Vegetarian Lentil and Sweet Potato Stew:
- Recommended Daily Intake: Men - 38 grams, Women - 25 grams
- Fiber Content: Approximately 14 grams per cup (cooked lentils and sweet potatoes)
- Nutrition: Lentils offer protein and fiber, while sweet potatoes add additional fiber and nutrients.

Desserts Recipes

1. Chia Seed Pudding with Berries:
Recommended Daily Intake: Men - 38 grams, Women - 25 grams
Fiber Content: Approximately 10 grams per 2 tablespoons of chia seeds (when mixed with liquid)
Nutrition: Chia seeds provide omega-3 fatty acids, and berries add antioxidants and vitamins.

2. Oatmeal Banana Cookies:
Recommended Daily Intake: Men - 38 grams, Women - 25 grams
Fiber Content: Approximately 3 grams per cookie (using oats and bananas)
Nutrition: Oats offer fiber, and bananas add natural sweetness and potassium.

3. Avocado Chocolate Mousse:
Recommended Daily Intake: Men - 38 grams,
Women - 25 grams
Fiber Content: Approximately 7 grams per half-cup
of avocado
Nutrition: Avocado provides healthy fats and fiber,
while cocoa powder adds a rich chocolate flavor.

4. Baked Apple with Cinnamon and Walnuts:
Recommended Daily Intake: Men - 38 grams,
Women - 25 grams
Fiber Content: Approximately 5 grams per medium-
sized apple
Nutrition: Apples offer fiber and natural sweetness,
and walnuts provide healthy fats.

5. Greek Yogurt Parfait with Granola and Fruit:
Recommended Daily Intake: Men - 38 grams,
Women - 25 grams
Fiber Content: Approximately 6 grams per cup of
Greek yogurt (without added sugars)
Nutrition: Greek yogurt provides protein, while
granola and fruit contribute fiber, vitamins, and
minerals.

6. Fruit Salad with Honey-Lime Dressing:
Recommended Daily Intake: Men - 38 grams,
Women - 25 grams
Fiber Content: Varies based on fruits used
Nutrition: Mixed fruits offer a variety of vitamins,
minerals, and fiber, and the honey-lime dressing adds
sweetness.

7. Bran Muffins with Raisins:
Recommended Daily Intake: Men - 38 grams, Women - 25 grams
Fiber Content: Approximately 5 grams per muffin (using bran)
Nutrition: Bran muffins offer fiber, and raisins add natural sweetness.

8. Coconut and Chia Seed Energy Bites:
Recommended Daily Intake: Men - 38 grams, Women - 25 grams
Fiber Content: Approximately 4 grams per serving (using chia seeds and coconut)
Nutrition: Chia seeds provide fiber, and coconut adds flavor and healthy fats.

9. Whole Wheat Banana Bread:
Recommended Daily Intake: Men - 38 grams, Women - 25 grams
Fiber Content: Approximately 2 grams per slice (using whole wheat flour and bananas)
Nutrition: Whole wheat flour offers more fiber than refined flour, and bananas provide natural sweetness.

10. Berry and Oat Crisp:
- Recommended Daily Intake: Men - 38 grams, Women - 25 grams
- Fiber Content: Approximately 6 grams per serving (using berries and oats)
- Nutrition: Berries offer antioxidants, and oats add fiber to this delicious crisp.

Snacks Recipes

1. Homemade Trail Mix:
Recommended Daily Intake: Men - 38 grams, Women - 25 grams
Fiber Content: Varies based on ingredients (nuts, seeds, dried fruits)
Nutrition: Nuts and seeds provide healthy fats and fiber, while dried fruits add natural sweetness.

2. Chickpea and Roasted Garlic Hummus:
Recommended Daily Intake: Men - 38 grams, Women - 25 grams
Fiber Content: Approximately 5 grams per 1/4 cup serving
Nutrition: Chickpeas offer protein and fiber, and garlic adds flavor.

3. Greek Yogurt with Berries and Almonds:
Recommended Daily Intake: Men - 38 grams, Women - 25 grams
Fiber Content: Approximately 6 grams per cup of Greek yogurt (without added sugars)
Nutrition: Greek yogurt provides protein, while berries and almonds contribute fiber and healthy fats.

4. Roasted Edamame:
Recommended Daily Intake: Men - 38 grams, Women - 25 grams
Fiber Content: Approximately 8 grams per cup (roasted edamame)
Nutrition: Edamame offers protein and fiber, and roasting adds a satisfying crunch.

5. Apple Slices with Peanut Butter:
Recommended Daily Intake: Men - 38 grams,
Women - 25 grams
Fiber Content: Approximately 4 grams per medium-
sized apple
Nutrition: Apples provide fiber and natural
sweetness, and peanut butter adds protein and
healthy fats.

6. Vegetable Sticks with Hummus:
Recommended Daily Intake: Men - 38 grams,
Women - 25 grams
Fiber Content: Varies based on vegetables (e.g.,
carrots, celery, bell peppers)
Nutrition: Hummus provides fiber and protein, and
vegetables add vitamins and minerals.

7. Dark Chocolate and Almond Clusters:
Recommended Daily Intake: Men - 38 grams,
Women - 25 grams
Fiber Content: Approximately 4 grams per ounce of
dark chocolate and almonds
Nutrition: Dark chocolate contains antioxidants, and
almonds provide fiber and healthy fats.

8. Whole Grain Crackers with Cheese:
Recommended Daily Intake: Men - 38 grams,
Women - 25 grams
Fiber Content: Varies based on crackers (choose
whole grain) and cheese
Nutrition: Whole grain crackers offer fiber, and
cheese provides protein and calcium.

9. Roasted Pumpkin Seeds:
Recommended Daily Intake: Men - 38 grams,
Women - 25 grams
Fiber Content: Approximately 5 grams per ounce of
roasted pumpkin seeds
Nutrition: Pumpkin seeds offer fiber, protein, and
healthy fats.

10. Yogurt and Berry Parfait with Granola:
- Recommended Daily Intake: Men - 38 grams,
Women - 25 grams
- Fiber Content: Approximately 5 grams per cup of
yogurt (without added sugars) and berries
- Nutrition: Yogurt provides protein, while berries
and granola contribute fiber, vitamins, and minerals.

Smoothies Recipes

1. Green Power Smoothie:
Recommended Daily Intake: Men - 38 grams,
Women - 25 grams
Fiber Content: Approximately 8 grams per serving
Nutrition: Spinach and kale provide fiber and
nutrients, while fruits add natural sweetness.

2. Berry Blast Smoothie:
Recommended Daily Intake: Men - 38 grams,
Women - 25 grams
Fiber Content: Approximately 10 grams per serving
Nutrition: Berries are rich in fiber and antioxidants,
and Greek yogurt adds protein.

3. Pineapple and Kale Tropical Smoothie:
Recommended Daily Intake: Men - 38 grams, Women - 25 grams
Fiber Content: Approximately 7 grams per serving
Nutrition: Pineapple and kale provide fiber and vitamins, and coconut water adds natural sweetness.

4. Mango and Chia Seed Smoothie:
Recommended Daily Intake: Men - 38 grams, Women - 25 grams
Fiber Content: Approximately 8 grams per serving
Nutrition: Mango offers fiber and a tropical flavor, while chia seeds provide omega-3 fatty acids.

5. Banana and Almond Butter Protein Smoothie:
Recommended Daily Intake: Men - 38 grams, Women - 25 grams
Fiber Content: Approximately 6 grams per serving
Nutrition: Bananas provide natural sweetness and fiber, and almond butter adds protein and healthy fats.

6. Avocado and Spinach Smoothie:
Recommended Daily Intake: Men - 38 grams, Women - 25 grams
Fiber Content: Approximately 9 grams per serving
Nutrition: Avocado offers healthy fats and fiber, and spinach provides additional nutrients.

7. Protein-Packed Blueberry and Oat Smoothie:
Recommended Daily Intake: Men - 38 grams, Women - 25 grams
Fiber Content: Approximately 7 grams per serving

Nutrition: Blueberries are rich in antioxidants and fiber, while oats add a hearty texture and additional fiber.

8. Strawberry and Banana Fiber Smoothie:
Recommended Daily Intake: Men - 38 grams, Women - 25 grams
Fiber Content: Approximately 6 grams per serving
Nutrition: Strawberries and bananas provide natural sweetness and fiber.

9. Cucumber and Kiwi Detox Smoothie:
Recommended Daily Intake: Men - 38 grams, Women - 25 grams
Fiber Content: Approximately 7 grams per serving
Nutrition: Cucumber adds hydration, while kiwi provides fiber and vitamin C.

10. Tropical Mango and Coconut Smoothie Bowl:
- Recommended Daily Intake: Men - 38 grams, Women - 25 grams
- Fiber Content: Approximately 9 grams per serving
- Nutrition: Mango and coconut milk create a tropical flavor, and toppings like granola and nuts add additional fiber and nutrients.

BENEFITS OF HIGH FIBER DIET

A high-fiber diet offers numerous health benefits, impacting various aspects of physical well-being. Here are some of the key benefits associated with incorporating a high-fiber diet into your lifestyle:

Improved Digestive Health:
1. Prevention of Constipation: Dietary fiber adds bulk to stool, softening it and promoting regular bowel movements, preventing constipation.
2. Prevention of Diverticular Disease: Adequate fiber intake may reduce the risk of diverticulosis and diverticulitis, conditions affecting the colon.

Weight Management:
- Increased Satiety: High-fiber foods take longer to chew and digest, promoting a feeling of fullness and reducing overall calorie intake, which can aid in weight management.

Blood Sugar Control:
- Stabilization of Blood Sugar Levels: Soluble fiber helps regulate blood glucose levels by slowing the absorption of sugar. This is particularly beneficial for individuals with diabetes or those at risk of developing diabetes.

Heart Health:

- Lowering Cholesterol Levels: Soluble fiber can help reduce LDL ("bad") cholesterol levels, contributing to cardiovascular health and lowering the risk of heart disease.
- Blood Pressure Regulation: Some studies suggest that a high-fiber diet may help maintain healthy blood pressure levels.

Prevention of Colorectal Cancer:

- Reduced Risk of Colorectal Cancer: A diet high in fiber, especially from whole grains, fruits, and vegetables, has been associated with a lower risk of developing colorectal cancer.

Healthy Weight Maintenance:

- Assistance in Weight Loss: High-fiber foods often require more chewing, leading to a slower eating pace. Additionally, fiber-rich foods are usually lower in calorie density, contributing to weight loss or weight maintenance.

Gut Microbiota Health:

Promotion of Beneficial Gut Bacteria: Fiber serves as a prebiotic, nourishing beneficial bacteria in the gut, which plays a crucial role in overall digestive and immune system health.

Reduced Risk of Type 2 Diabetes:
- Lowered Risk of Type 2 Diabetes: High-fiber diets have been associated with a reduced risk of developing type 2 diabetes, possibly due to improved blood sugar control and insulin sensitivity.

Healthy Aging:
- Cognitive Health: Some research suggests that a diet rich in fiber may contribute to better cognitive function and a lower risk of age-related cognitive decline.

Inflammation Reduction:
- Anti-Inflammatory Effects: Some types of fiber, particularly found in fruits, vegetables, and whole grains, have anti-inflammatory properties that may help reduce inflammation in the body.
- It's important to note that individual responses to dietary changes may vary, and it's always advisable to consult with a healthcare professional or a registered dietitian for personalized advice. Additionally, it's crucial to stay adequately hydrated when increasing fiber intake to prevent potential digestive discomfort.

Certainly! Here are some of the best sources of high-fiber foods along with their approximate fiber contents per serving:

Beans and Legumes:
- Black beans (cooked, 1 cup): ~15 grams of fiber
- Lentils (cooked, 1 cup): ~15.6 grams of fiber
- Chickpeas (cooked, 1 cup): ~12.5 grams of fiber

Whole Grains:
- Quinoa (cooked, 1 cup): ~5.2 grams of fiber
- Oats (cooked, 1 cup): ~4 grams of fiber
- Brown rice (cooked, 1 cup): ~3.5 grams of fiber

Fruits:
- Raspberries (1 cup): ~8 grams of fiber
- Pear (medium, with skin): ~5.5 grams of fiber
- Apple (medium, with skin): ~4.4 grams of fiber
- Banana (medium): ~3.1 grams of fiber
- Avocado (1 cup, sliced): ~10 grams of fiber

Vegetables:
- Artichoke (1 medium): ~6.7 grams of fiber
- Broccoli (1 cup, cooked): ~2.4 grams of fiber

- Brussels sprouts (1 cup, cooked): ~3.3 grams of fiber
- Carrot (1 cup, raw): ~3.6 grams of fiber
- Spinach (1 cup, cooked): ~6.7 grams of fiber

Nuts and Seeds:
- Chia seeds (1 ounce): ~10.6 grams of fiber
- Flaxseeds (1 ounce): ~7.6 grams of fiber
- Almonds (1 ounce): ~3.5 grams of fiber
- Pumpkin seeds (1 ounce): ~5.2 grams of fiber

Cereals:
- Bran flakes (3/4 cup): ~7 grams of fiber
- Shredded wheat (2 biscuits): ~6 grams of fiber
- All-Bran (1/2 cup): ~10 grams of fiber
- Quinoa flakes (1/2 cup): ~5 grams of fiber

HOW TO ADD MORE FIBER TO YOUR DIET

Adding more fiber to your diet is a beneficial way to improve your overall health and support proper digestion. Here are some practical tips to increase your fiber intake:

Choose Whole Grains:
Opt for whole grain options such as whole wheat bread, brown rice, quinoa, oats, and whole grain pasta instead of refined grains.

Eat More Fruits and Vegetables:
Aim to include a variety of fruits and vegetables in your meals. Add berries, apples, pears, oranges, leafy greens, carrots, and other colorful produce to your diet.

Include Legumes and Beans:
Incorporate beans, lentils, chickpeas, and other legumes into your meals. They can be added to salads, soups, stews, or used as a meat substitute in certain dishes.

Snack on Nuts and Seeds:
Enjoy nuts (almonds, walnuts, etc.) and seeds (chia, flax, sunflower) as snacks or add them to yogurt, salads, or smoothies.

Choose High-Fiber Cereals:
Select cereals that are high in fiber and low in added sugars. Look for options with whole grains and bran.

Eat More Whole Fruits Instead of Fruit Juices:
Whole fruits contain more fiber than fruit juices. Choose whole fruits like apples, oranges, and berries as snacks or desserts.

Add Vegetables to Every Meal:
Incorporate vegetables into your breakfast, lunch, and dinner. Add spinach to your omelets, include a side of roasted vegetables, or mix them into pasta dishes.

Include Fiber-Rich Snacks:
Choose snacks that are high in fiber, such as air-popped popcorn, whole fruits, raw vegetables with hummus, or a handful of nuts.

Use Whole Grains in Cooking:
Replace refined grains with whole grains in your cooking. For example, use brown rice instead of white rice, whole wheat flour instead of white flour, and whole grain breadcrumbs in recipes.

Gradually Increase Fiber Intake:
Sudden increases in fiber can cause digestive discomfort. Gradually increase your fiber intake and drink plenty of water to help your digestive system adjust.

Read Food Labels:
Check food labels for fiber content. Look for products with higher fiber content and fewer added sugars.

Stay Hydrated:
- Drink plenty of water throughout the day, especially when increasing your fiber intake. Water helps move fiber through the digestive tract and prevents constipation.
- Remember that it's essential to balance fiber intake with adequate hydration to support proper digestion. If you have any specific dietary concerns or health conditions, consider consulting with a healthcare

professional or a registered dietitian for personalized advice.

SYMPTOMS OF EATING TOO MUCH FIBER

While a high-fiber diet is generally beneficial for most people, consuming excessive amounts of fiber can lead to certain symptoms and digestive issues. Here are some common symptoms of eating too much fiber:

Gastrointestinal Discomfort:
Consuming excessive fiber can lead to bloating, gas, and abdominal discomfort. This is especially true if your body is not accustomed to a high-fiber diet.

Diarrhea:
Eating too much fiber, particularly insoluble fiber found in some whole grains and certain fruits and vegetables, can lead to loose stools and diarrhea.

Constipation:
In some cases, an abrupt increase in fiber intake without sufficient water intake can lead to constipation. It's important to balance fiber with an adequate amount of fluids.

Dehydration:
Fiber absorbs water, and if you don't increase your fluid intake along with a high-fiber diet, it may lead to dehydration.

Nutrient Malabsorption:
Excessive fiber intake can interfere with the absorption of certain minerals, such as calcium, iron, zinc, and magnesium. This can be a concern, especially if your diet relies heavily on fortified foods.

Stomach Upset:
Some individuals may experience stomach upset, including nausea or a feeling of fullness, when they consume too much fiber in a short period.

Intestinal Blockage:
Though rare, excessive fiber intake without adequate fluid consumption could potentially lead to intestinal blockage in extreme cases.

Interference with Medication:
High-fiber foods can interfere with the absorption of certain medications. If you are on medication, consult your healthcare provider about the potential interactions.

Allergic Reactions:
In rare cases, individuals may be allergic to specific high-fiber foods, leading to allergic reactions such as itching, hives, or swelling.

Weight Loss or Inadequate Nutrition:
A diet extremely high in fiber, especially if it leads
to reduced overall food intake, can potentially result
in weight loss and inadequate nutrition.

PROCESS TO REDUCED HIGH FIBER SYMPTOMS

If you're experiencing symptoms due to a high-fiber
diet, there are several steps you can take to alleviate
discomfort and gradually adjust to increased fiber
intake. Here's a process to help reduce high-fiber
symptoms:

Gradual Increase:
If you've recently increased your fiber intake and are
experiencing symptoms, consider scaling back
temporarily. Gradually introduce fiber-rich foods to
give your digestive system time to adapt.

Stay Hydrated:
Ensure you are drinking enough water. Fiber absorbs
water, and adequate hydration is crucial for proper
digestion. Aim for at least 8 cups (64 ounces) of
water per day, and more if you're physically active.

Balanced Diet:
Maintain a balanced diet with a mix of soluble and
insoluble fibers. Soluble fibers, found in oats, beans,
and fruits, can be gentler on the digestive system than
some insoluble fibers found in certain vegetables and
whole grains.

Identify Problematic Foods:
Identify specific foods that might be causing discomfort. Some people are more sensitive to certain types of fiber or particular high-fiber foods. Experiment with different sources of fiber to see what suits you best.

Cooking Methods:
Experiment with different cooking methods. Sometimes lightly cooking or steaming vegetables can make them more digestible than consuming them raw.

Consider Fiber Supplements:
If your symptoms persist, consider talking to a healthcare professional about using fiber supplements. They can provide a controlled amount of fiber, and you can gradually increase the dose as your body adjusts.

Probiotics:
Probiotics, found in certain foods or as supplements, can help promote a healthy balance of gut bacteria and may aid in digestion. Consult with a healthcare professional before starting a probiotic regimen.

Monitor Portion Sizes:
Pay attention to portion sizes, especially when it comes to high-fiber foods. Overeating, even healthy foods, can lead to digestive discomfort.

Limit Gas-Producing Foods:
Some high-fiber foods can produce gas during digestion. Limit intake of gas-producing foods, such as beans and cruciferous vegetables, until your digestive system adjusts.

Seek Professional Advice:
If symptoms persist or if you have concerns about your digestive health, consult with a healthcare professional or a registered dietitian. They can provide personalized advice based on your health history and dietary preferences.

MEAL PLANNING TIPS FOR HIGH FIBER

Meal planning for a high-fiber diet involves incorporating a variety of nutrient-rich foods that are naturally high in fiber. Here are some tips to help you create a balanced and fiber-rich meal plan:

Include a Variety of Whole Grains:
Choose whole grains like brown rice, quinoa, whole wheat pasta, barley, and oats. These grains are higher in fiber compared to their refined counterparts.

Load Up on Vegetables:
Make vegetables a centerpiece of your meals. Include a variety of colorful vegetables in salads, stir-fries, soups, and side dishes. Aim for different types to get a mix of soluble and insoluble fiber.

Incorporate Legumes and Beans:
Include beans, lentils, and chickpeas in your meals. These are excellent sources of fiber and can be added to salads, stews, soups, or used as a meat substitute in various dishes.

Choose High-Fiber Fruits:
Opt for fruits that are rich in fiber, such as berries, apples, pears, oranges, and kiwi. Eat them as snacks, add them to yogurt, or include them in smoothies.

Select Lean Protein Sources:
Choose lean protein sources like poultry, fish, tofu, eggs, and legumes. Pairing lean proteins with high-fiber foods can create satisfying and nutritious meals.

Incorporate Nuts and Seeds:
Add nuts and seeds, such as almonds, chia seeds, flaxseeds, and sunflower seeds, to salads, yogurt, or as a topping for whole grain dishes. They provide additional fiber and healthy fats.

Choose High-Fiber Snacks:
Snack on whole fruits, raw vegetables with hummus, yogurt with berries and granola, or a handful of nuts. These snacks can contribute to your daily fiber intake.

Plan Balanced Meals:
Create balanced meals that include a mix of carbohydrates, proteins, and healthy fats. This helps keep you satisfied and provides a broad range of nutrients.

Experiment with Fiber-Rich Recipes:
Look for or create recipes that incorporate high-fiber ingredients. Experiment with different cooking methods and flavor combinations to keep your meals interesting.

Stay Hydrated:
Drink plenty of water throughout the day. Fiber absorbs water, and adequate hydration helps prevent constipation and supports optimal digestion.

Read Labels:
When purchasing packaged foods, check the nutrition labels to identify the fiber content. Choose

products with higher fiber content and lower added sugars.

Prep and Cook in Batches:
Plan and prepare meals in advance, especially high-fiber grains, beans, and vegetables. Having these ingredients ready makes it easier to put together nutritious meals during the week.

Use Herbs and Spices:
Enhance the flavor of your high-fiber meals with herbs and spices instead of relying on excessive salt, sugar, or unhealthy fats.

Gradual Changes:
If you're not used to a high-fiber diet, introduce fiber-rich foods gradually to give your digestive system time to adjust.

Fruits:

- Apples
- Bananas
- Berries (blueberries, strawberries, raspberries)
- Oranges
- Pears
- Kiwi
- Mangoes
- Avocado
- Grapefruit
- Grapes

Vegetables:

- Spinach
- Kale
- Broccoli
- Cauliflower
- Carrots
- Bell peppers
- Sweet potatoes
- Brussels sprouts
- Zucchini
- Cabbage

Whole Grains:

- Quinoa
- Brown rice
- Oats (steel-cut or rolled oats)

- Barley
- Whole wheat pasta
- Farro
- Bulgur
- Millet
- Buckwheat
- Whole wheat bread

Legumes:
- Lentils (green, brown, red)
- Chickpeas
- Black beans
- Kidney beans
- Pinto beans
- Split peas
- Navy beans
- Edamame
- Hummus

Nuts and Seeds:
- Almonds
- Walnuts
- Chia seeds
- Flaxseeds
- Sunflower seeds
- Pumpkin seeds
- Pistachios
- Sesame seeds
- Hemp seeds
- Nut butters (almond butter, peanut butter)

Dairy and Alternatives:

- Greek yogurt (unsweetened)
- Cottage cheese
- Almond milk
- Soy milk
- Flavored yogurt with added fiber

Proteins:

- Chicken breast
- Turkey breast
- Salmon
- Tofu
- Tempeh
- Eggs

Cereals and Breakfast Items:

- High-fiber cereal (check labels for fiber content)
- Whole grain granola
- Oat bran
- Bran flakes
- Whole grain pancakes or waffles

Dried Fruits:

- Raisins
- Apricots
- Prunes
- Dates
- Figs

Condiments and Extras:

- Olive oil
- Balsamic vinegar
- Honey or maple syrup (as sweeteners)
- Herbs and spices (to add flavor without added calories)
- Salsa (tomato-based)

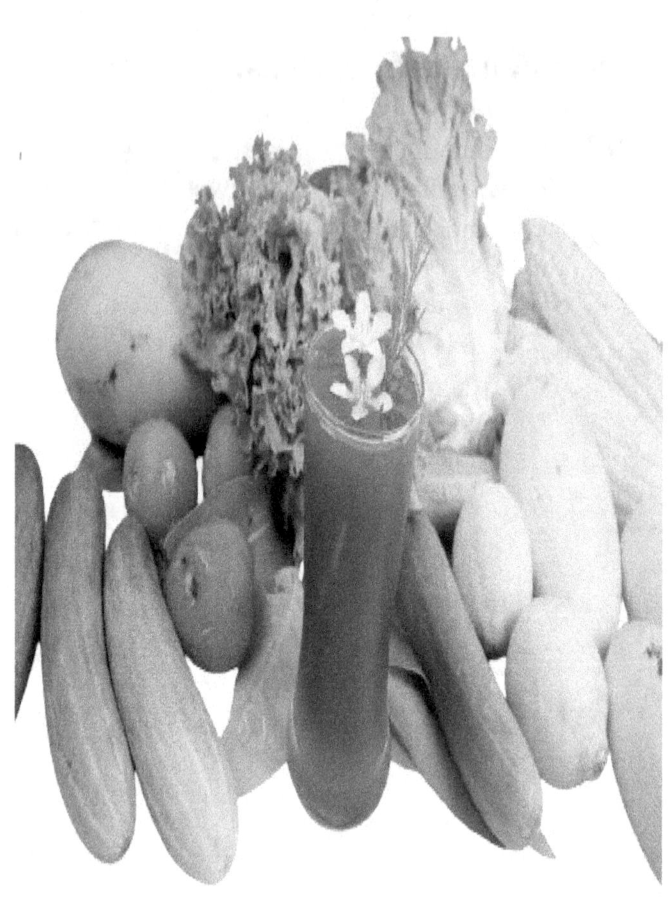

CONCLUSION

In conclusion, incorporating a variety of high-fiber foods into your daily diet is a simple yet powerful way to enhance your overall health and well-being. The diverse selection of fruits, vegetables, whole grains, legumes, nuts, and seeds included in this high-fiber food list offers not only an abundance of fiber but also a myriad of essential nutrients.

The benefits of a high-fiber diet extend beyond promoting digestive health. Fiber plays a crucial role in managing weight, regulating blood sugar levels, lowering cholesterol, and supporting heart health. By embracing the foods on this list, you are not only nourishing your body with fiber but also providing it with vitamins, minerals, antioxidants, and other bioactive compounds that contribute to a robust and resilient system.

As you explore and incorporate these high-fiber options into your meals, remember that dietary changes should be approached with balance and consideration for individual health needs. Consulting with a healthcare professional or a registered dietitian can provide personalized guidance on how to optimize your fiber intake based on your specific health goals.